A Present for Paul

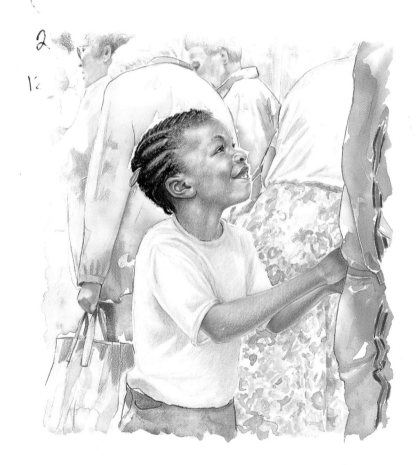

First published in hardback in Great Britain by
HarperCollins Publishers Ltd in 1996
First published in paperback by Picture Lions in 1996
7 9 10 8 6
ISBN: 0 00 664160 1
Picture Lions is an imprint of the Children's Division,
part of HarperCollins Publishers Ltd.
Text copyright © Bernard Ashley 1996
Illustrations copyright © David Mitchell 1996
The author and illustrator assert the moral right to be identified as the
author and illustrator of the work.
A CIP catalogue record for this title is available from the British Library.
The HarperCollins website address is: www.fireandwater.com
Printed and bound in Singapore

A Present for Paul

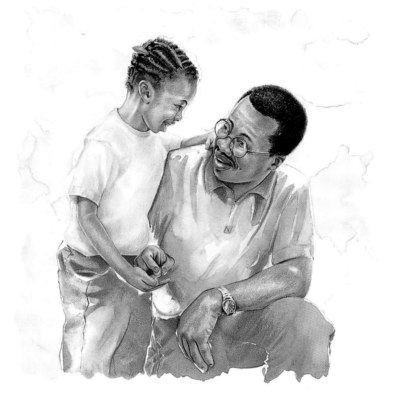

BERNARD ASHLEY

ILLUSTRATED BY DAVID MITCHELL

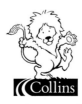

Collins

An imprint of HarperCollinsPublishers

It was Saturday and baby Paul was hurting badly with a new tooth coming through.

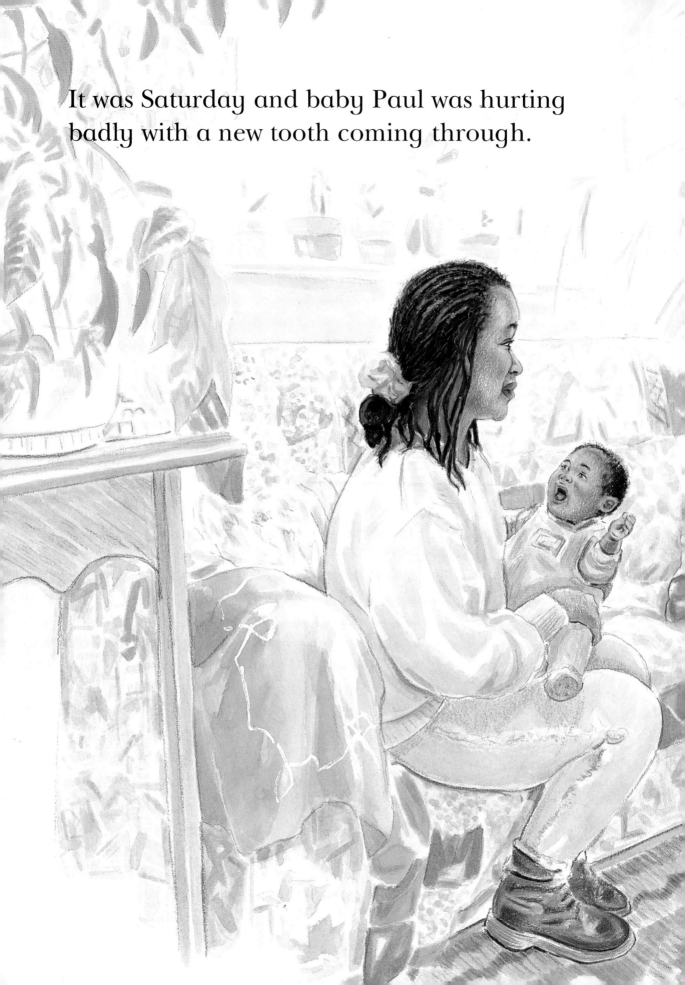

Pleasure's dad said he'd do the shopping alone
– unless his big girl wanted to help.
"But you'd better stay close," he told her.
"That market's a busy old place today."

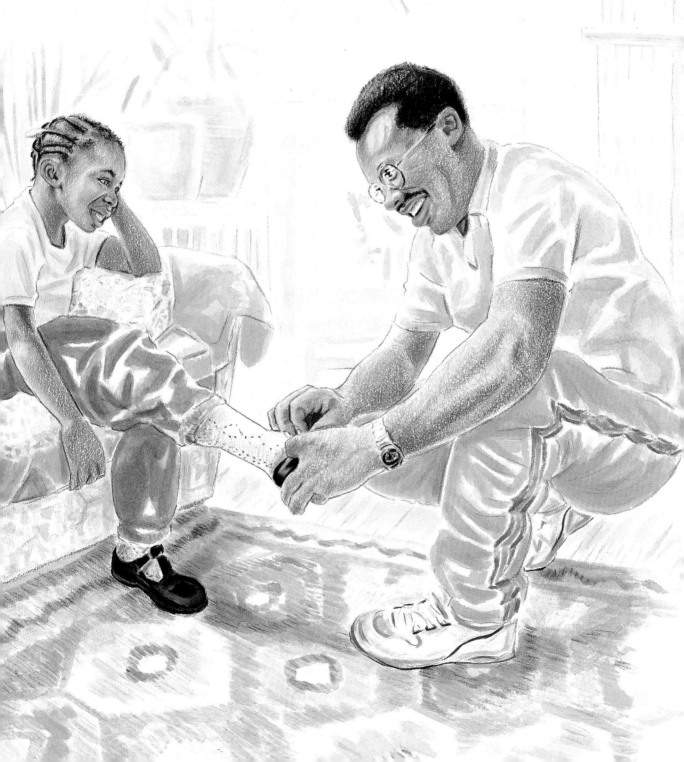

On the top of the bus going to market Pleasure showed what she'd got in her hand.

"A pound for a present for Paul," she said. But her dad was busy checking his list.

At the market the stalls looked bright from above: loads of good fun like a fair.

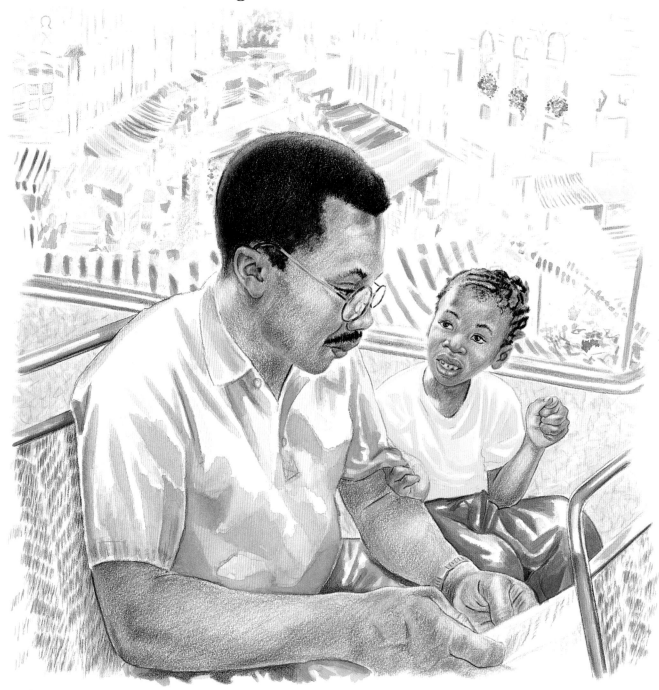

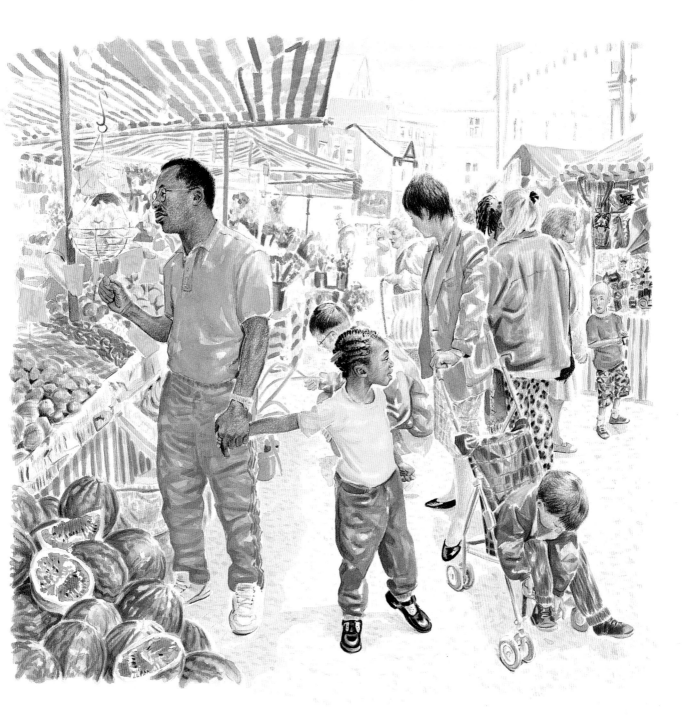

But it was all bustle and bags when they got off
the bus. And Dad with all that shopping to do.
   "Vegetables," he said, holding her tightly.
And he bought chillies, potatoes and beans.
But Pleasure was eyeing the children's stall.
   "I want to get something for Paul."

"And I'm after fish while it's fresh," Dad said. He let Pleasure pick out their supper, but she didn't give it too much of a look. Paul wouldn't thank them for haddock, but he'd like a rattle to shake!

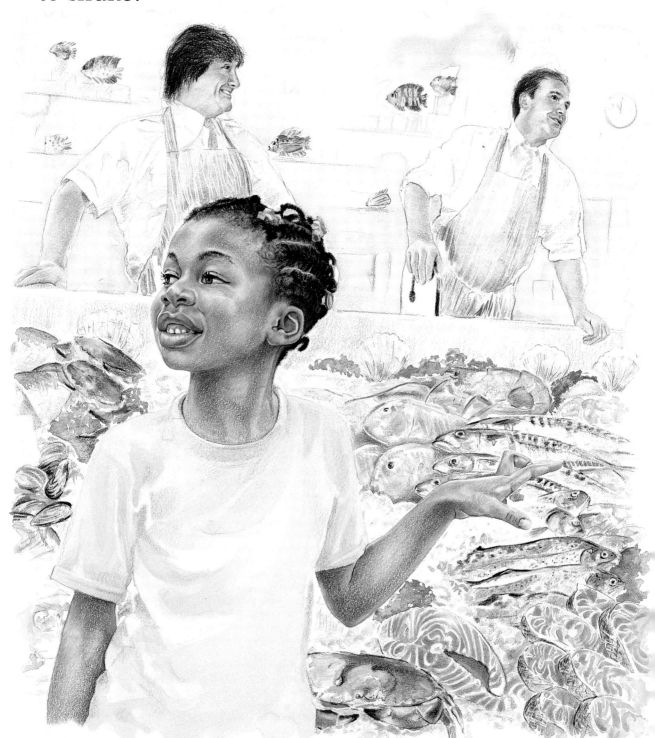

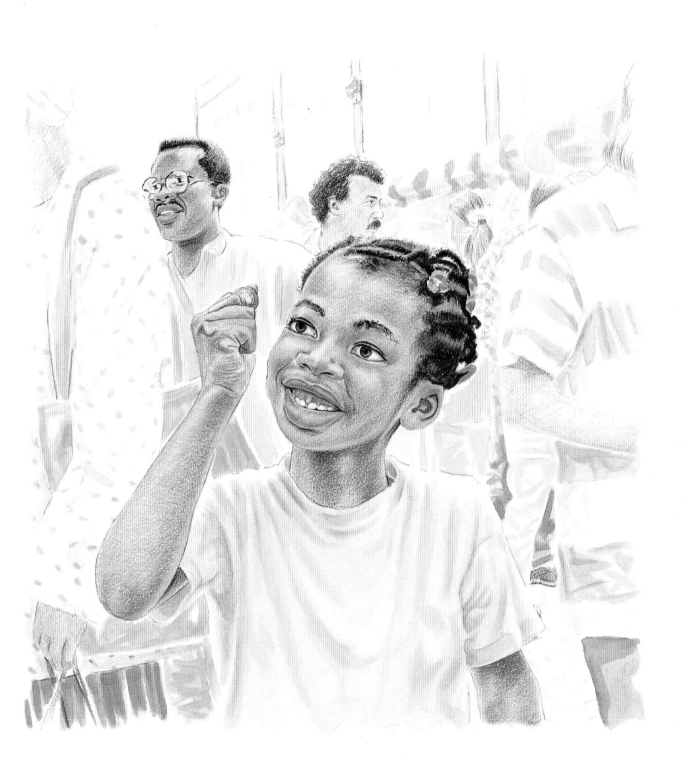

And her hand went straight to her pocket when her father let go to pay. Because over there was a teething ring – just right for the baby to bite.

She twisted round for permission with a pleasure smile on her face. She was thinking how pleased the baby would be – but the smile was wiped off in a flash.

"Dad…!"

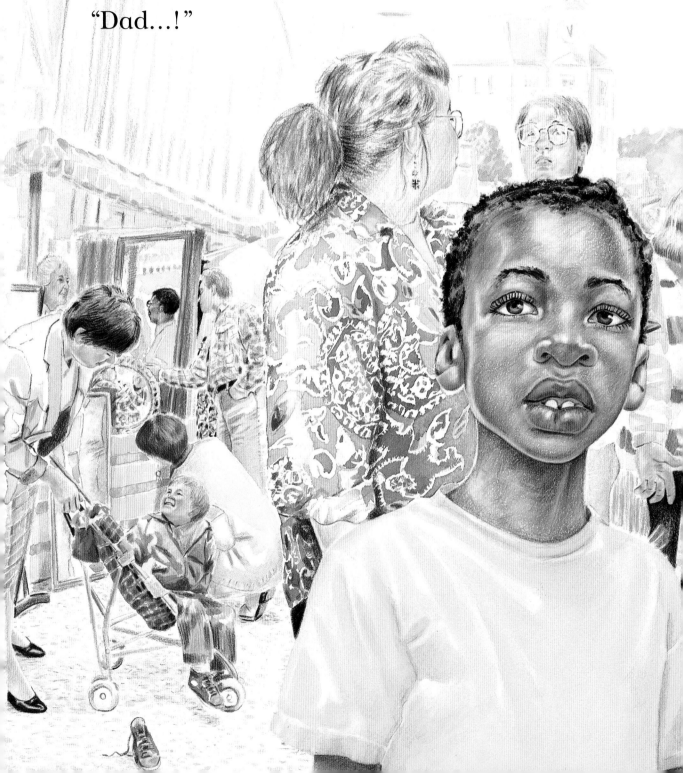

Because her dad wasn't there any more!

He wasn't there?

Where was he? She'd only just turned round, how could he have gone so quick? She twisted back the other way – but he wasn't there either, only strangers' legs and their coats and their bags.

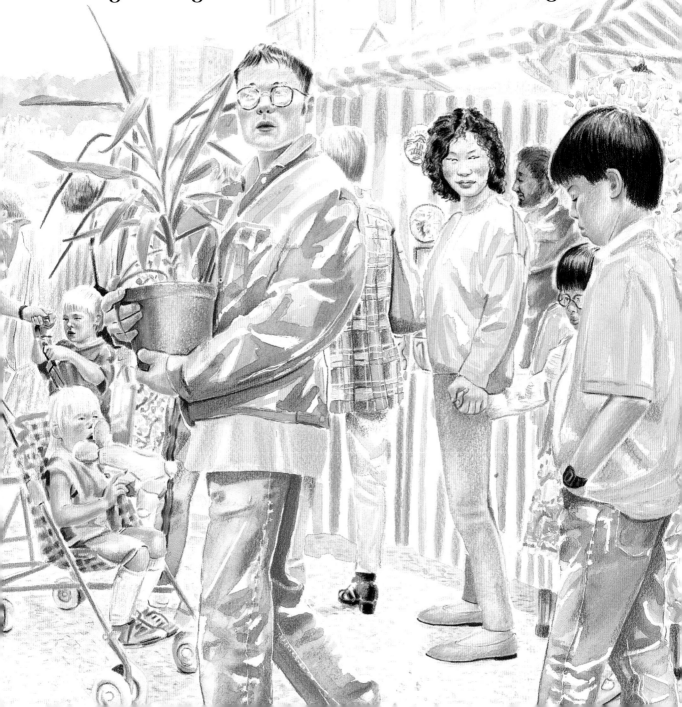

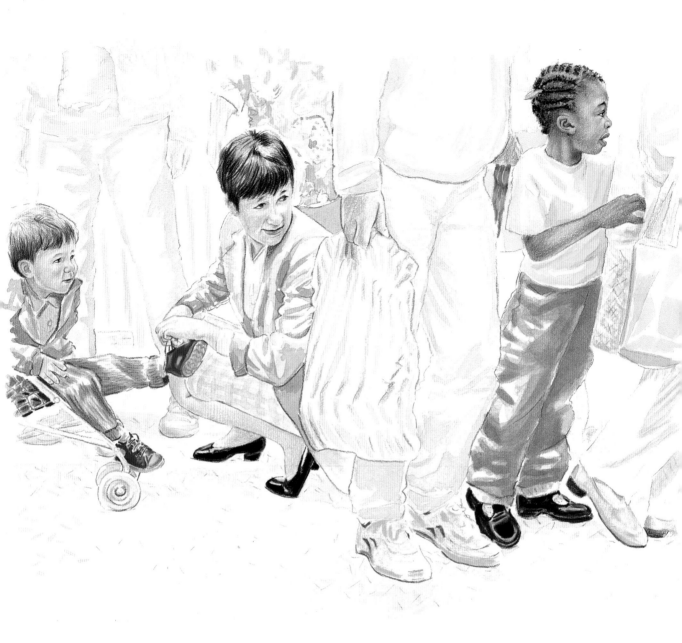

There was everyone else, but no sign of him!
Her stomach did a head over heels – but he
always said she was his big girl, so she wasn't
going to get scared!

She pushed through the legs, she stood on her toes. He couldn't have gone very far.

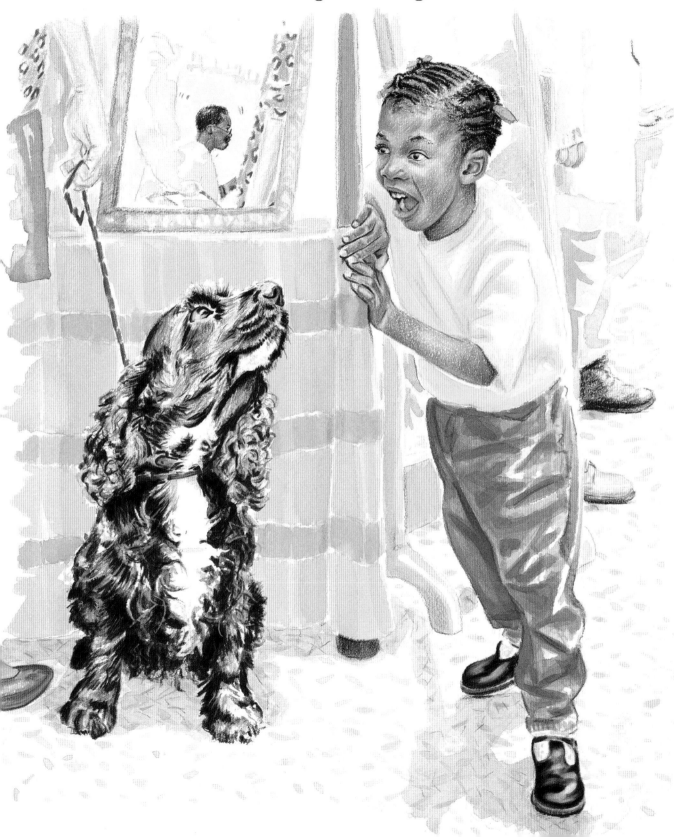

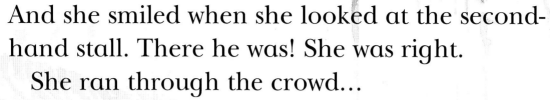

And she smiled when she looked at the second-
hand stall. There he was! She was right.
She ran through the crowd...

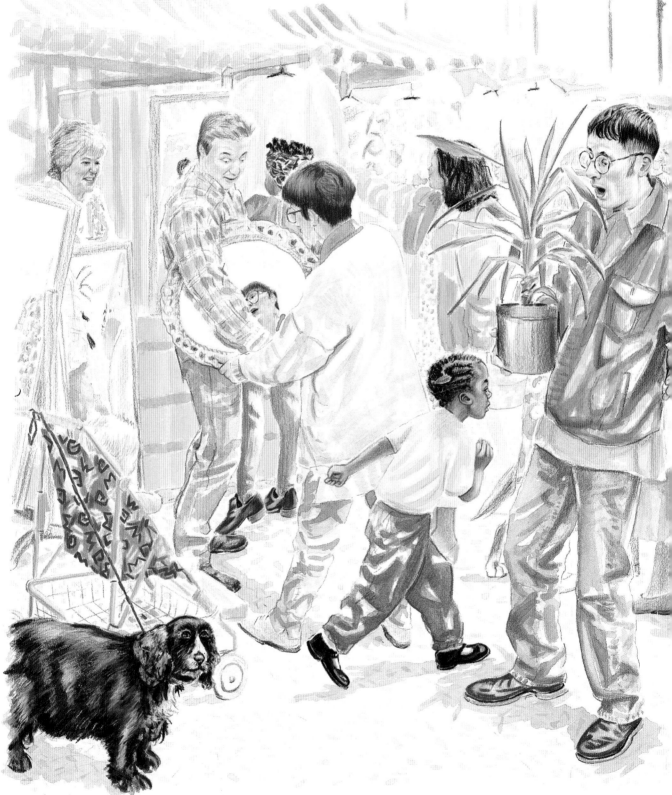

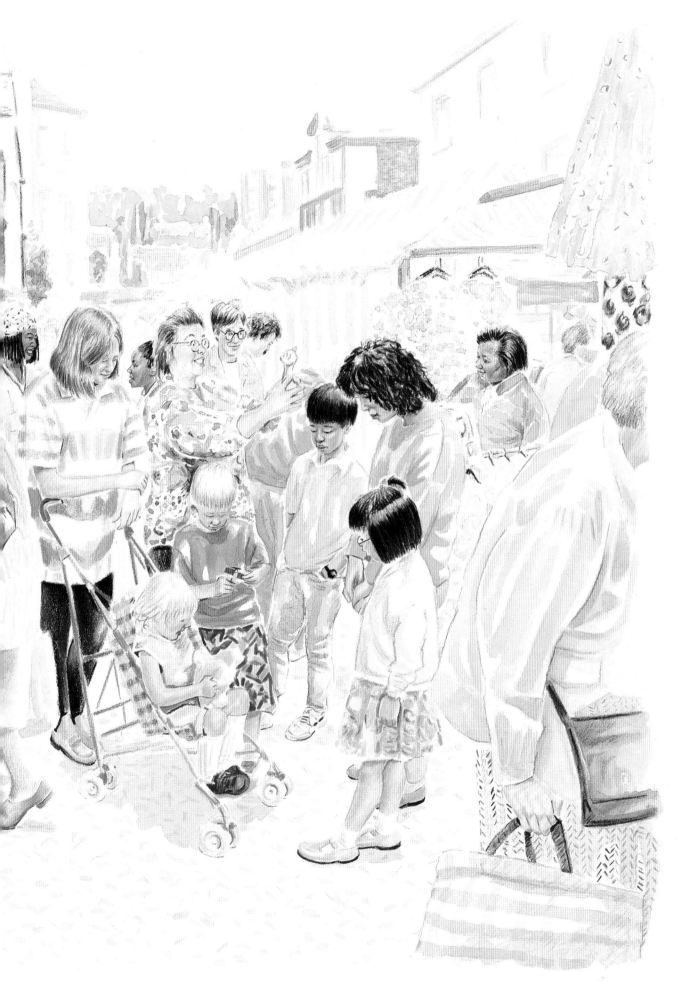

...and grabbed hard at his tracksuit.
But – up close the striping was different,

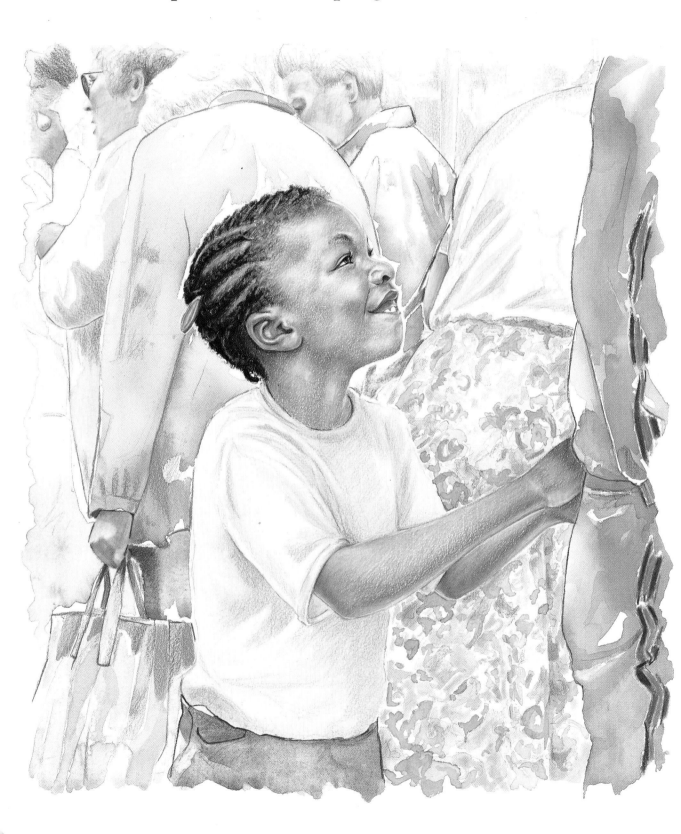

and so was the face staring down.

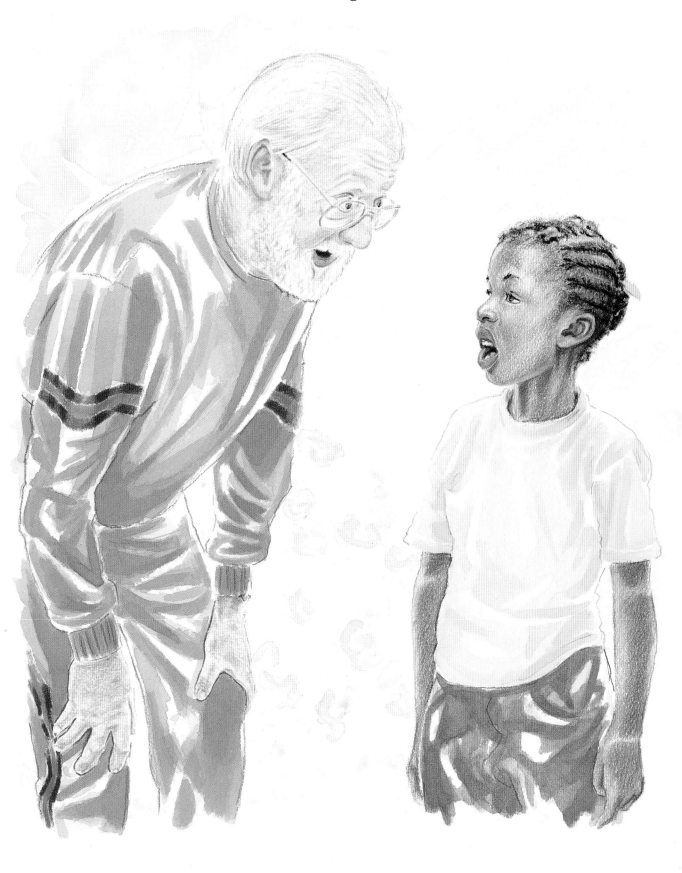

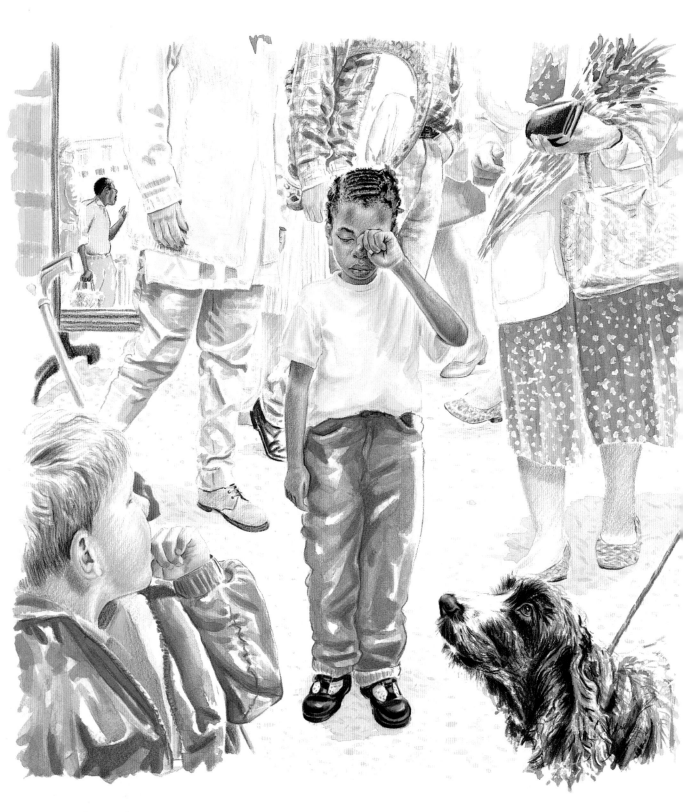

Now Pleasure *did* feel frightened, like the only child in the world.

"She's lost!" someone said. "The poor little mite!"
And people started calling her, "Love".

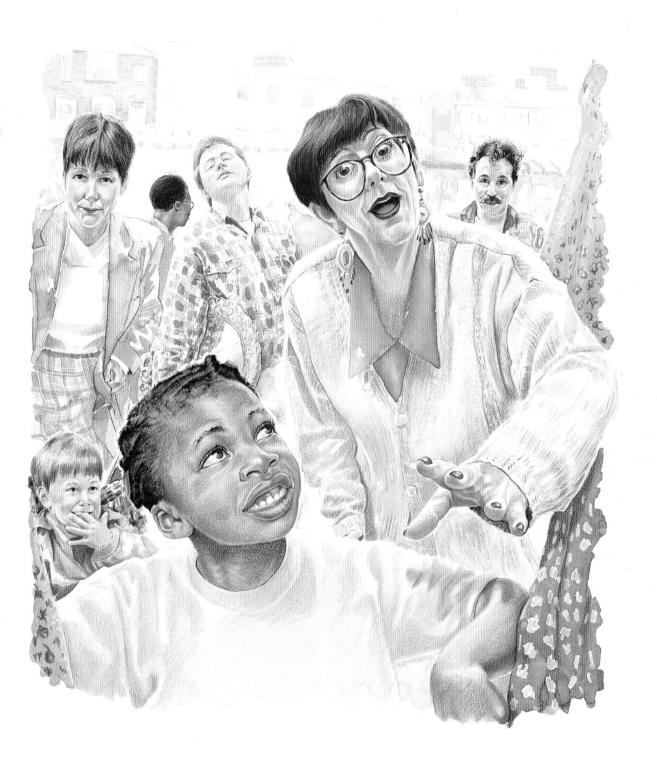

A whole staring ring of them crowding her in,

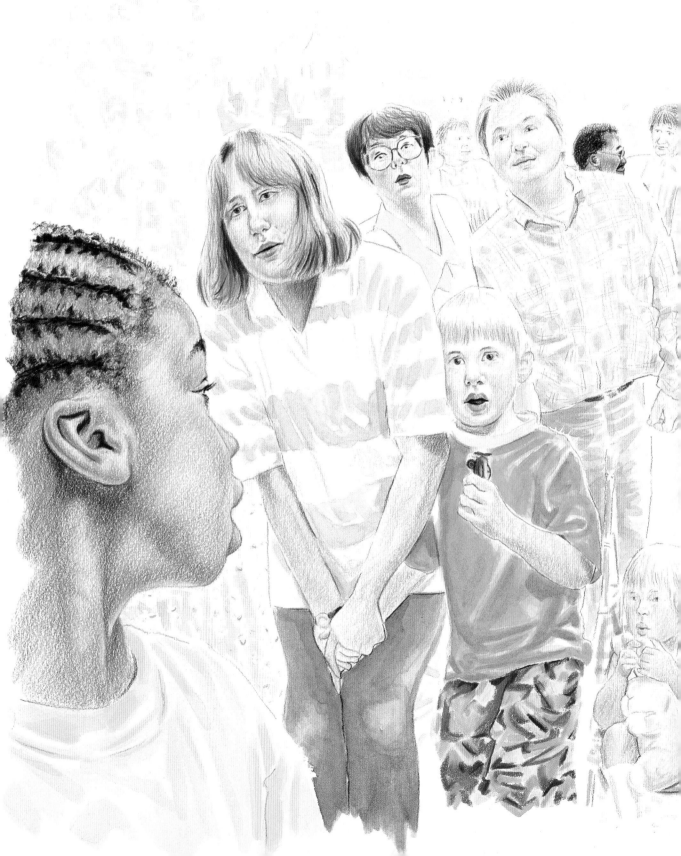

like trapping a wounded bird.

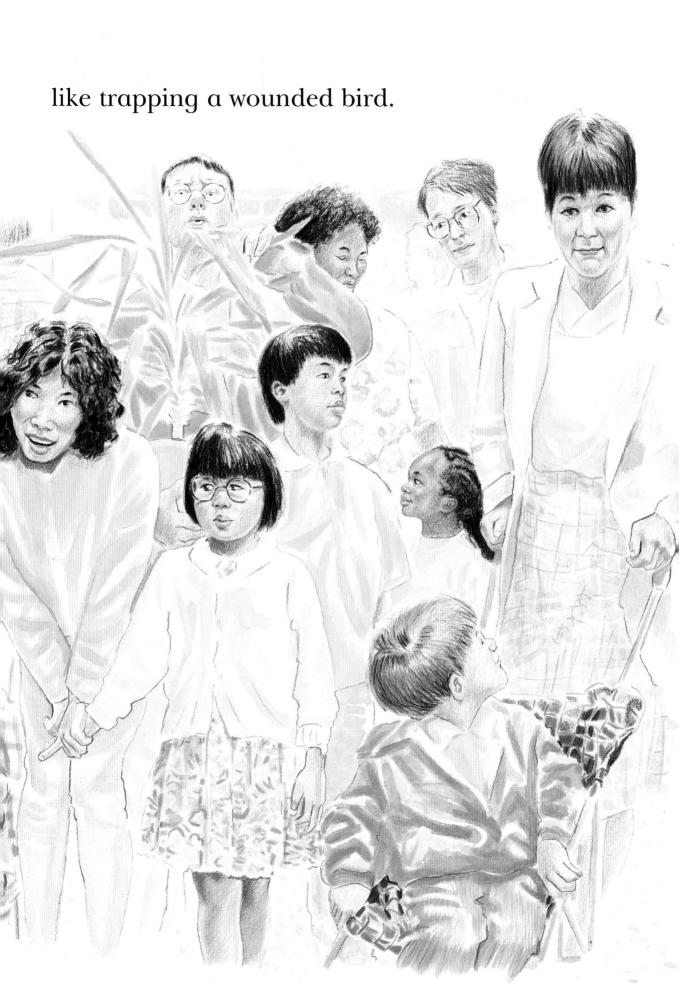

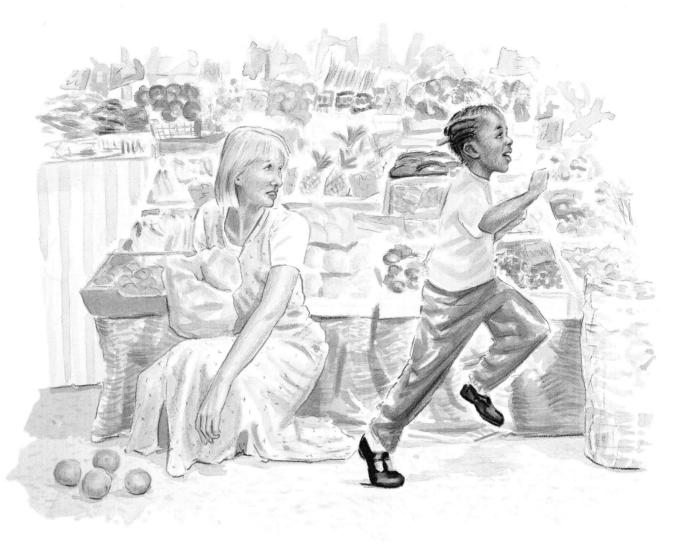

She turned and she
ran, she didn't know
where, but away from
their hands and their
shouts. He'd got to
be somewhere! He'd
got to! And he'd be
going mad looking
for her.

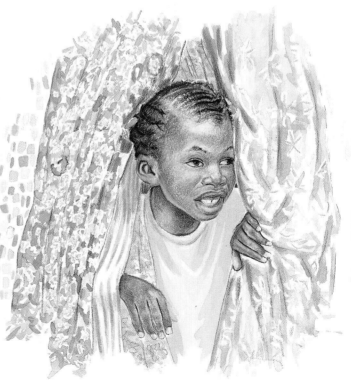

She shouted, "DAD!" like a Tannoy, and chased through the stalls in a state.

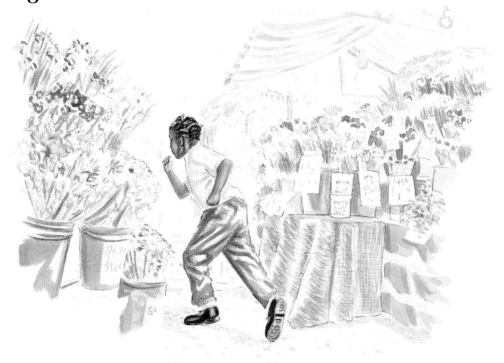

Through dresses and fruit and flowers and bags.

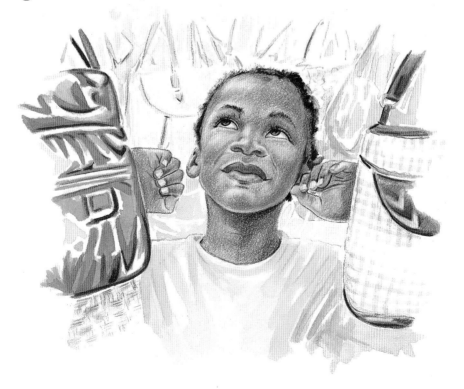

Till she came shouting in panic round one last stall, to the fish – where he was counting his change.

"What's the matter with you, girl?"

He hadn't missed her at all.

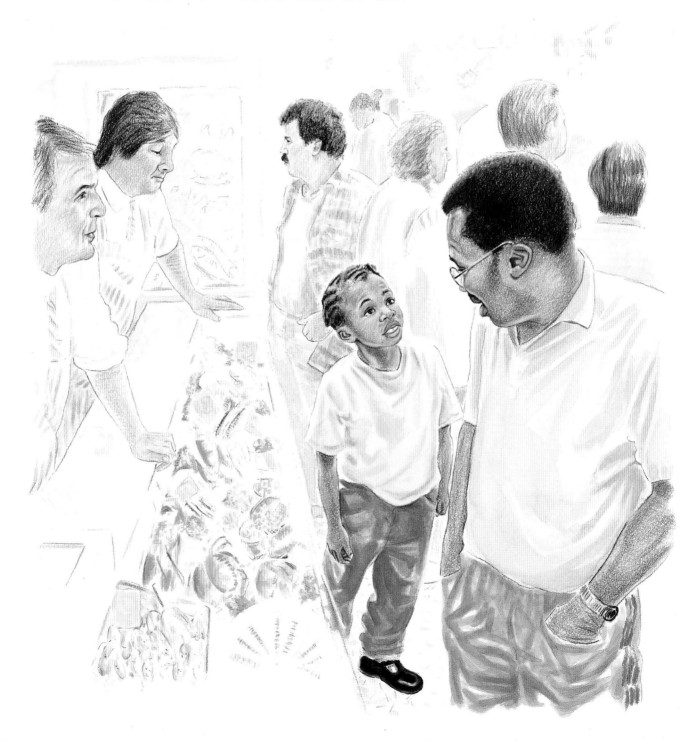

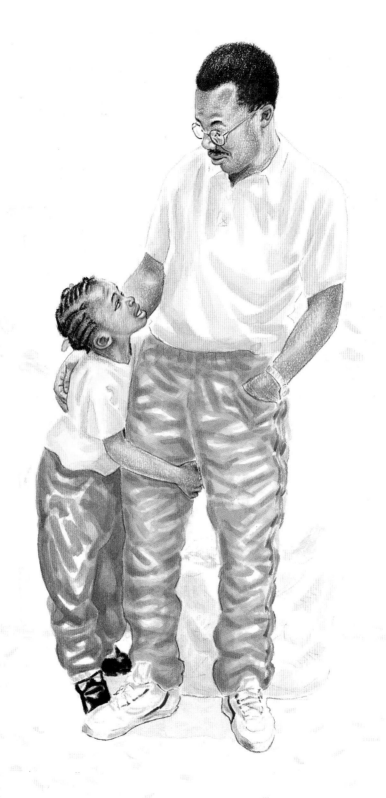

But she grabbed him in case she lost him again.
"Where *were* you!" she cried into his clothes.
"Where was I? I haven't budged an inch."

And then he spoke softly to calm her down,
tried to get her thinking about something else.
  "Did you choose what you're getting for
Paul," he asked, "before you lost sight of me?"

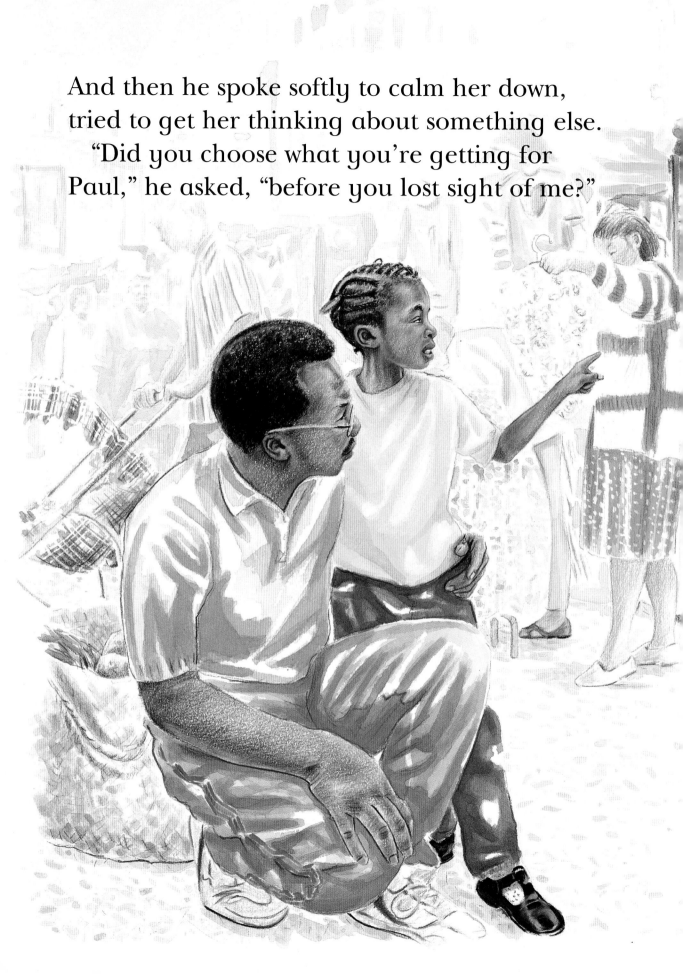

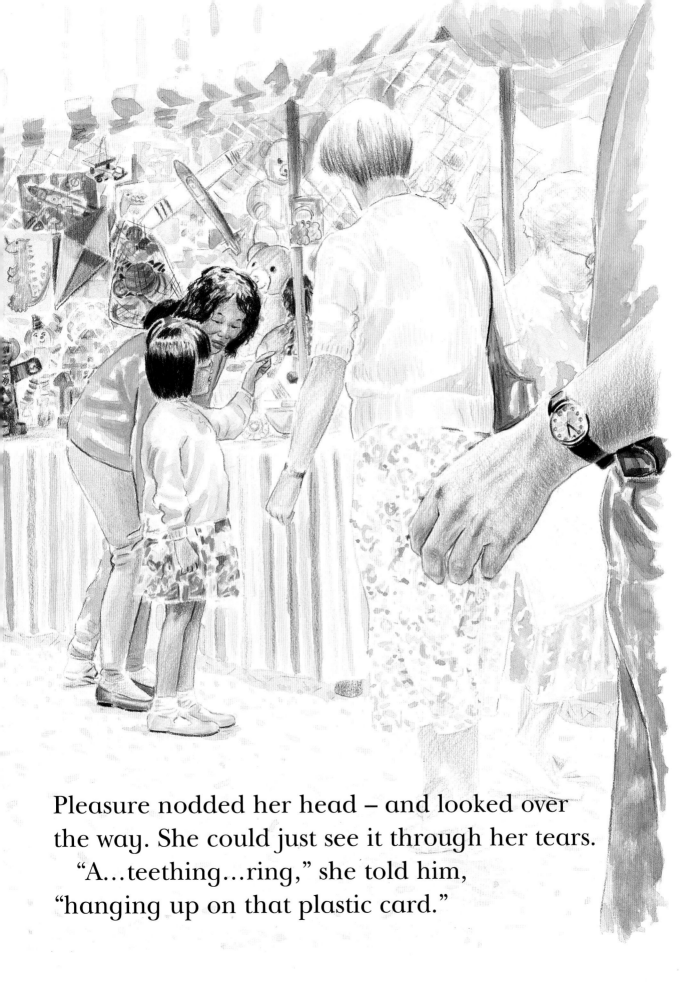

Pleasure nodded her head – and looked over
the way. She could just see it through her tears.
  "A…teething…ring," she told him,
"hanging up on that plastic card."

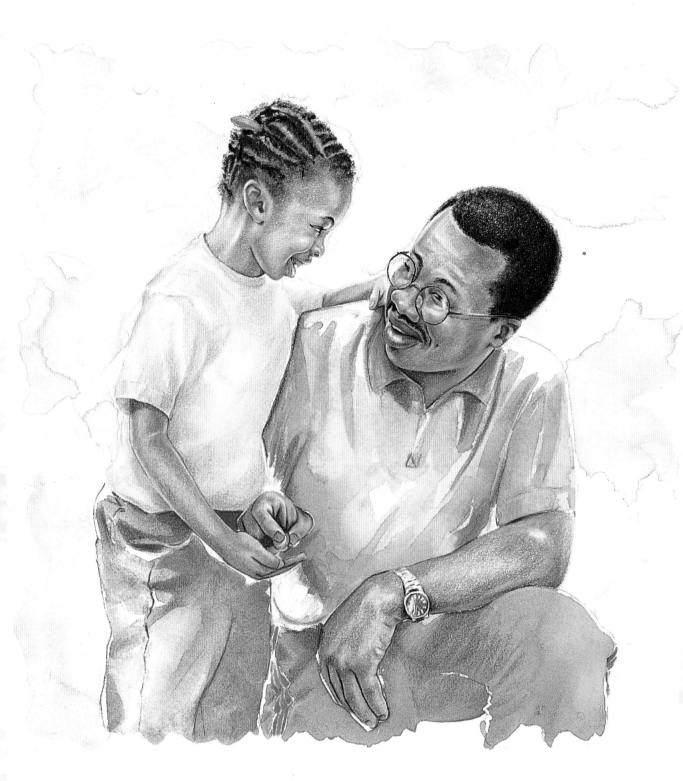

"That's nice. And what about something for somebody else? For a bit of comfort, after a scare."

He put his hand in his pocket. He was going to give her a treat.

Pleasure looked over at the stall again, not feeling like his big girl at all. There were toys and dolls and books and games.

"But I've been a bit of a baby," she told Dad, "I'd better have that dummy over there!"

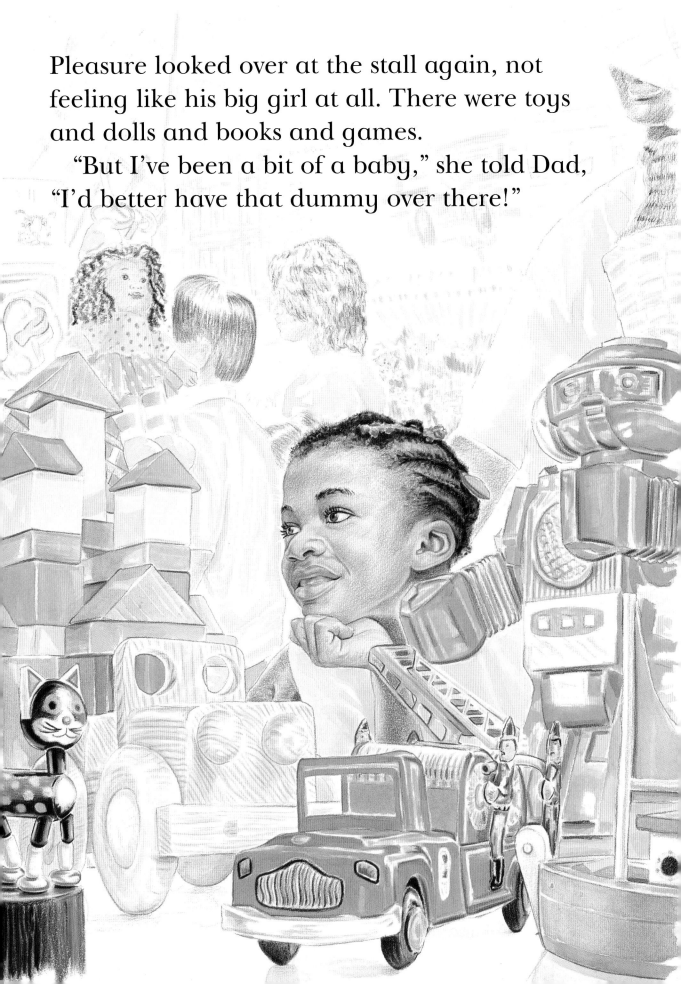

And his smile made everything right.

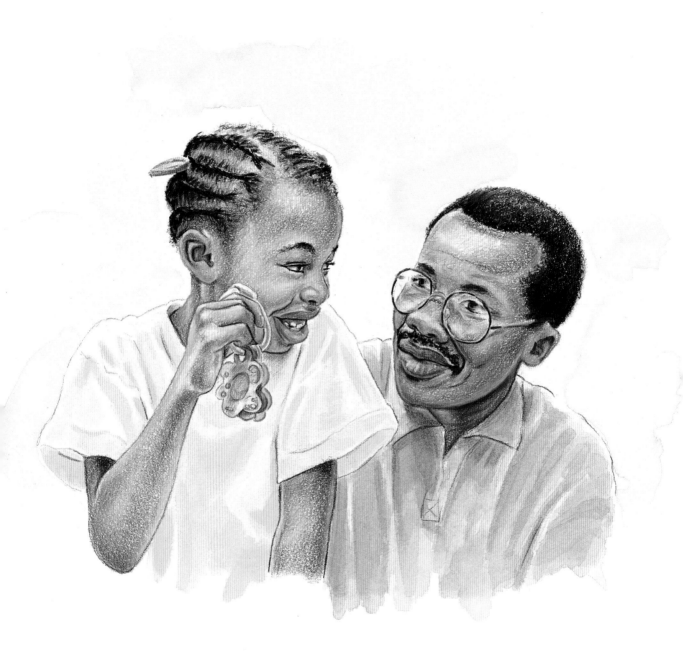

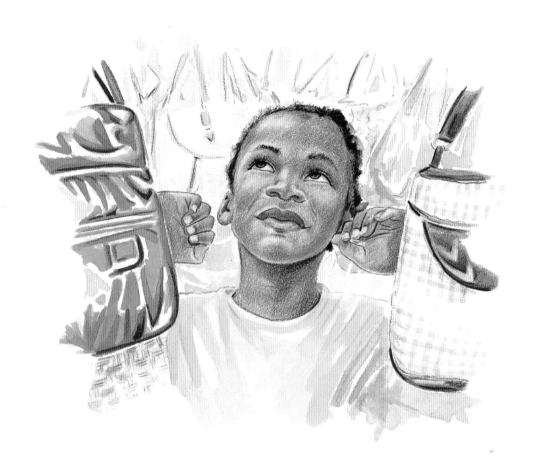